CBD

What you should know and how it is applied

FlyGirl

ISBN: 9781657059108

ISBN: 9781657059108

CONTENTS

FLYGIRLS MESSAGE:

2019 I was brave enough to publish my first book. A completely different topic (Wind Therapy – A book about female riders worldwide).

But there is more about me:

Over the past years – as we all get older – lol - we feel our bodies.

Some of us suffer from diseases, overcame cancer, ….and some take meds and don`t even get a lot relieve.

There are alternatives to all this drugs.
But don`t get me wrong: the alternatives are NO miracle cure!

The Alternatives have the ability to bring you some relieve and yes, even a better life quality after a while.

And they don`t work the same with every disease or person.

So please, read, be responsible and don`t be afraid to seek the help of a professional when you are unsure.

And don`t forget to check out your county/State laws before you buy and use CBD!

1 INTRODUCTION

Hardly any other plant has been so controversially discussed in recent years as the hemp plant.
But hemp is not only the intoxicating herb for smoking, but rather a very diverse plant.
In addition to all the different fields of application, the active ingredient cannabidiol has fortunately been given particular attention in recent years.
Many new and old findings do not promise miracles, but for many people relief and alleviation.

The hemp plant was already cultivated several thousand years ago in Asia.
Because: Hemp is a very versatile plant.
The fiber can be used for the manufacturing of clothing and ropes and the seeds are a component of nutrition.
Already over 500 years ago, there were first records about the medical use of the hemp plant.
Also, the drug ingredients of the hemp plant were already used in pre-Christian times in many religious rites.
Many people only know hemp as a "drug".
Many medical applications of hemp first had to be rediscovered again.
The Europeans who travelled to Asia in the 17th century first reported on "Indian hemp". This was cannabis with a very high THC content.
However, it took until 1830 for a German professor to report in detail about the medical uses of hemp for the first time.

The first publication on the medical use of cannabis, which has received widespread attention, was written by the Scottish physician Sir William Brooke O`Shaughnessy. He stayed in India for a long time and managed to gather a lot of information about the medical and popular use of the hemp plant.
His reports on the use of cannabis tinctures (in rheumatism, delirium tremens, cramps, tetanus) found some attention and prompted him to perform studies on animals and humans.

Gradually more doctors in Europe and America began to use cannabis in medicine. And the positive reports of relief and healing successes increased.
Also astonishing was the range of clinical pictures where cannabis was used successfully:

- Migraine
- Depression
- Chronic Pains
- Arthritis
- Muscle Cramps
- Asthma
- Stomach Pains
- Sleeplessness
- Menstrual Cramps
- Promotion of contractions
- ...

At the end of the 19th century, cannabis products were a recognized medicine in America and Europe. Even the first pharmaceutical companies produced preparations.
As development and industrialization progressed, the curiosity to research the active ingredients of cannabis grew.
THC for example was already "identified" at the beginning of the 20th century, but only in 1964 was it possible to determine a chemical structure.
Today we know that the hemp plant contains about 489 different components.
There are 70 different Phyto cannabinoids in the group alone.
The best known are THC, CBD, CBN.
THC is the component of the hemp plant that has an intoxicating and therefore psychoactive effect.
CBD, on the other hand, is not psychoactive or intoxicating, but can be used effectively and safely in therapy and medicine due to its anti-schizophrenic, anti-inflammatory and anti-epileptic properties. The experience reports of affected persons are all positive and more and more people are experiencing relief from long-standing disease patterns by taking CBD.

After this rough overview, it is worth taking a closer look at CBD, its active ingredients, how it works in individual cases and how it is best applied.
A natural remedy that is fortunately becoming more and more popular and therefore more accepted.

So, let's get to know and understand CBD a little better!

2 WHAT IS A CANNABIDIOL? WHAT IS CBD?

From a purely chemical point of view, CBD ($C_{21}H_{30}O_2$) is a cannabidiol.
This means that its active ingredients are hardly psychoactive.
In the hemp plant it occurs predominantly as CBD carboxylic acid and is obtained by various extraction processes.
The CBD extracts obtained in this way can now be used in many different ways. Used as a remedy and painkiller, it achieves very good results.
CBD was used as a remedy thousands of years ago, but in recent years it has fortunately experienced some kind of revival.
The reason for this is certainly the search of many people for alternative healing or relief possibilities.
Especially patients with chronic pain who have been taking strong medication for years, are often amazed how well CBD actually helps.
Often the doses of painkillers must be increased over the years, which leads to further strain on the body, side effects and drug dependence.
CBD is the natural alternative!
Today it is possible (from a chemical point of view), to identify and explore the many active ingredients and components of the cannabis plant.
In the past, people just realized: the application is good for me.
Today, of course, all this information is analyzed, and the curiosity of the researchers makes further research possible.
Through all these old and new insights, e.g. the mode of action of CBD can also be determined much more accurately.

Hardly anyone can say today that he / she has not heard CBD at least once before.
Because sometimes you have the impression in recent years that CBD is

omnipresent.
It has become a trend.
For many people it is just a "lifestyle product".
But very few of these "trend users" know exactly what CBD is and what to consider when using CBD.

3 LEGALITY OF CBD

First of all, it is important to get rid of some rumors and find out exactly to what extent CBD is legal or illegal.

And this is not an easy topic at all!

The widespread statement: "CBD is legal. Only THC is illegal" looks very tempting and good at first sight.

Also, you will read again and again: CBD contains no THC, so has no intoxication and is therefore legal.

This statement is basically correct in theory and on paper, but the user/consumer is still obliged to inform himself/herself beforehand.

The definition within the EU (European Union) is: CBD is legal, but every country within the EU has its own guidelines and laws.

This is similar to the USA: each state has its own laws and regulations about CBD.

Example:

You are on vacation in Switzerland and discover a hemp cigarette at a kiosk (and they have a real good hemp cigarette).

Curious, you inquire and learn, yes, it is a legal product, because it is a CBD hemp cigarette and therefor legal.

It doesn`t have an intoxicating but a relaxing effect.

In spite of the high price (about $ 25/pack) and because you are on holiday, you buy a pack.

After one week you start the journey home and still have some cigarettes in the pack, which of course should travel home with you. You're legal.

And this is where the "country trap" snaps shut:

In Switzerland, it is legal for CBD products to still contain a small THC share of up to 1%.

This value is also the basis to produce hemp cigarettes.

You must therefore assume that in the worst case and in order to preserve the legality of the product, the hemp cigarette from Switzerland can have a value of 0.999 % THC.
You travel home to Germany via Austria.
In the EU there are no border controls anymore, but you can be stopped by mobile customs units and any time!
In Austria, the maximum permitted THC content for CBD products is 0.3 %.
Means: an import of the Swiss hemp cigarettes to Austria (even if it is only a transit country) is already illegal.
Arriving in Germany - the cigarettes are still in your luggage, because you only drove a short distance through Austria - you have to know: also in Germany the CBD cigarettes from Switzerland are illegal.
The limit value THC in Germany is 0.2%.

This is just one example of how different the borders between legality and illegality of CBD are in the 3 neighboring countries in Europe.

Within the USA there are different state laws too.
So please inform yourself before you start using CBD in your state.
When you plan to travel within the US with CBD products which still might contain a small amount of THC, please check the state laws!

But there are many more points to consider.

As an example:

The rule for CBD products in Germany is: CBD is only legal if it is not psychoactive!
Since CBD products are cannabidiol and they are not psychoactive - i.e. have no consciousness changing effects (like THC) - CBD oil is legal for the time being.
Only: these products should be as pure as possible, because they may only have a THC content of 0.0005 %!
Exactly this information should also be shown on the CBD products.
But reality shows: there are no information's about THC content on the majority of CBD product.
Please don`t assume they are all THC free!

In Germany it is only allowed to sell products with this extremely low THC content, but in case of doubt every buyer is responsible to check this himself.

In Germany, the legal position of CBD is still being disputed.
Since 2016 the following regulation applies:
As long as the "marketing promise" for CBD promises no medical benefit, no healing power, it is not subject to prescription and can be freely purchased like dietary supplements.

4 PREPARATION OF CBD AND IT`S ACTIVE INGRIDIENT CANNABIDIOL

The CBD sold in our latitudes is made from the female hemp crop.
The female hemp crop naturally contains much less THC (cannabinoid).
In total, a hemp plant has more than 60 different cannabidiols and more than 480 active ingredients.
THC and cannabidiol are the most important active ingredients.

Cannabinoids (THC) have psychoactive agents.
Cannabidiole (CBD) are hardly psychoactive.

<u>Manufacturing</u>
The CBD extract is obtained by distillation.
The cannabinoids are triggered during the maceration of hemp flowers in alcohol.
The macerate is then mixed with hemp seed oil.

In Germany and Austria, only hemp plants that are subject to a special approval process are used for CBD production.
The cultivation of the approx. 80 hemp varieties approved in Europe is reserved only for certified farmers.
The natural THC content of the varieties used, must be detectable below 0,2 % THC.
Only varieties classified in this way may be sown.
Why is this so important?
A low THC value of the plant guarantees that the THC content of the end product is neutralized by the high-dose CBD.

Only female hemp plants are able to form hemp flowers.

As a result, female plants carry a much higher number of active substances (CBD, THC, CBN) than male plants.

<u>Active substance Cannabidiol</u>

As already mentioned, there are more than 60 different cannabidiols.

By far not all modes of action are known or have been scientifically researched and proven.

Among the effects that have been scientifically researched and proven so far are the following:

CBD stimulates (like capsaicin in sharp chilies, etc.) the so-called vanilloid receptor. This stimulation is said to have a pain-inhibiting effect.

CBD forfeits an increased release of neurotransmitters (noradrenaline, adrenaline).

In animal experiments the inflammation parameters were reduced by CBD. CBD binds to receptors that have anti-inflammatory effects.

Cannabidiols are strong radical scavengers and have very good cell protective properties.

This is part of the existing scientific statement but does not cover the full spectrum of CBD active substances.

How does CBD work?

The most effective way to consume CBD is in the form of extracted oil, because the ingredients contained in the oil are quickly and easily absorbed by the body.

Besides the mentioned ingredients, important cannabidiols are contained in CBD oil. These cannabidiols have different modes of action:

CBD = inflammations of all kinds, chronic pain, migraine attacks, cramps, arthritis, epilepsy, killing malignant tumor cells

CBC = cell renewal, anti-inflammatory and analgesic effect

CBDA = antiemetic effect against breast cancer, other cancers, nausea

CBG = antibacterial effect (may be stronger than usual antibiotics)

CBN = for acute states of anxiety and panic

Furthermore, you can find:

Vitamins

trace elements and minerals (calcium, magnesium, iron, zinc, phosphorus, manganese)

Omega 3 & 6

Gamma linolenic acid

Carotenoids
Chlorophyll

CBD has a very broad spectrum of action.

Why does CBD work so well in the body?
The human body has an ECS (Endo Cannabinoid System) and various receptors.
The ECS works together with other connection points in the body.
This means that it is responsible for how well the immune system works, how the sleep behavior is, and how intense you feel pain.

The ECS system is activated by the intake of CBD oil.
A previously irritated immune system can function normally again, sleep becomes deep and good, pain is relieved.

Since clinical studies are unfortunately still lacking, there are only attempts to explain why CBD works so well in the body.
It is assumed that CB2 receptors interact with CBD.
These CB2 receptors are responsible for the body's immune system, inflammatory reactions and pain.

The National Center for Biotechnology Information in the USA published its first results in 2017.
In summary, it was concluded that joint pain and joint inflammation (arthritis) can be alleviated. Long-term nerve damage and neuropathic pain can be prevented.

Chronic pain patients have hope that they can be helped in this way. Of course, this hope alone has a positive influence on the psyche of the patient, too.

Furthermore, allergies and diabetes can be prevented, possibly even be stopped.
It is hoped that there will soon be medical and scientific studies that will provide accurate insights into the exact mode of action of cannabidiol.

5 CBD APPLICATION AREAS

CBD products have been experiencing a boom in recent years.
This is mainly due to the fact that many users report soothing and improving effects.
Often these are people who are chronically ill and, despite orthodox medical treatment and conventional medication, have hardly been able to improve their state of health.
These people are very open when it comes to alternative ways of relief.
From their experience reports and those of the accompanying therapists, it is now possible to compile a good overview.

<u>Sleeplessness</u>
Tension, not being rested, reduced performance, ...are often the result of insomnia or a sleep that is interrupted again and again by waking up.
Sleeping pills are often the only help to sleep through the night.
But if you don't want to resort directly to sleeping pills, CBD oil is a very good alternative.
In contrast to sleeping pills, it is considered to be free of side effects.
Correctly dosed one can sleep through again and is more relaxed in the morning.

<u>Acne</u>
Acne is no longer just a problem with teenagers. More and more adults have skin problems and are therefore prone to acne.
The antibacterial and anti-inflammatory effect of CBD helps to reduce the skin's fat content. In this way acne can be fought in the long run.

<u>Smoking Cessation</u>
Initial studies have shown that smokers who inhaled CBD oil instead of

smoking a cigarette have less appetite for cigarettes over time. Within the study, this led to a 40 % reduction in cigarette consumption.

Overload, nervousness, stress
The calming effect of CBD oil has a relaxing and calming effect on overload, nervousness, stress and also on anxiety.

Diabetes
CBD oil has shown good effects in diabetes prevention.
Unfortunately, there are only studies on this with mice: overweight mice that received CBD did not develop diabetes despite having the same eating habits and still being overweight.

Multiple Sclerosis
Again, tested on mice, CBD was able to provide relief.
Already after ten days of CBD intake, mice showed an improvement of their general condition. Even the mobility became better again.

In the case of diabetes and multiple sclerosis, there are still many studies to be carried out, but the initial successes are very promising and give cause for hope.
Many diabetes and MS patients already rely on CBD.

Crohn's disease and fibromyalgia
Crohn's disease patients who already take CBD oil regularly report a significant improvement of the disease.

In the case of fibromyalgia, the symptoms were significantly alleviated.
In both cases, the anti-inflammatory effect of CBD is responsible for these positive developments.

Asthma and Allergies
Since CBD oil has been shown to stimulate the immune system and have anti-inflammatory effects, it is very helpful in diseases such as asthma and allergies.
The misdirected immune system that can cause asthma is successfully treated with CBD oil.

Allergies break out when the body's own defenses are no longer sufficient in a weak immune system. These are strengthened by CBD and the risk of developing allergies is reduced.

Alzheimer's and dementia

These degenerative diseases of the brain gives off a harmful protein that damages the nerve tracts. It causes the brain to slowly die.

Unfortunately, no scientific results from human studies are yet available, but the results from animal experiments raise great hopes.

Arthritis/Arthrosis

Arthrosis is a degenerative disease of the human cartilage tissue.

The anti-inflammatory effect of CBD oil can relieve arthritis.

Arthritis is the precursor to osteoarthritis.

By alleviating already in the stage of arthritis and inhibiting inflammation, not so much cartilage is broken down.

This does not necessarily lead to osteoarthritis. There is also the possibility that the course of the disease may be attenuated overall.

If the cartilage is already degraded, CBD oil cannot restore it!

It can only help relieve the pain.

BSE

BSE is not curable. It is a contagious, serious and fatal disease.

If one encounters promises of palliation or healing with CBD oil, this is not credible!

Nausea

If you have nausea, you may be reluctant to consume an oily liquid.

But the strong calming effect of CBD oil would be worth a try.

But you can take CBD oil drop by drop.

Epilepsy

For those suffering from epilepsy, the following advice applies: before trying out CBD on your own, please consult a doctor first and discuss the subject of CBD with him or her.

There are some "sensational videos" on the Internet.

Please never follow the instructions given there!

Epilepsy can lead to a life-threatening condition.

It's not worth risking your life through experiments!

Obesity and overweight

In case of a change in diet, CBD is a useful aid due to its appetite-restraining effect.

Taking CBD alone cannot cause weight loss.

In combination with a carbohydrate poor diet and plenty of exercise, however, it can have a supportive effect.

<u>Hepatitis</u>
If you suspect you have an inflammation of the liver (hepatitis is an infection of the liver), the first step is to see a doctor.
An appropriate diagnosis is important.
Hepatitis needs intensive medical treatment and self-experiments with CBD oil are strenuous.

<u>Cancer</u>
CBD is NOT a cure for cancer!
However, the effects of chemotherapy can be alleviated by taking CBD.
Attention: do not take CBD oil during chemotherapy!
It is well known that it has an appetite - controlling effect and cancer patients in an ongoing treatment have a high need for calories to give their body the strength to fight the malignant cancer cells with all their might.
<u>Nervous disorders</u>
For Parkinson's disease and other nerve diseases, CBD oil in a higher concentration can provide good support.

<u>Rheumatism</u>
Here, too, one can only rely on experience reports.
Rheumatism patients report a relief of pain as a result of taking CBD.

<u>Sepsis</u>
In the case of blood poisoning (sepsis) the treatment is usually exhausting.
CBD oil can calm the nerves and strengthen the immune system.
Sepsis itself is not alleviated.
This can only be done with the help of the doctor.

<u>Addictions</u>
CBD oil is not an addictive remedy.
However, it helps in the weaning phase because it can alleviate the pressure of addiction and combat emerging depressions.

6 HOW TO FIND A GOOD AND PURE CBD PRODUCT?

First, an important hint:
CBD products can now be easily found and purchased on the Internet with a single click. The offer is almost overwhelming.
But how can you, as an interested person or sick person who is concerned with the subject, find out whether it is also a good and pure CBD product?

Hemp shops that offer CBD products are already almost nationwide.
Qualified personnel can certainly answer many questions here.

BUT: the contents of all these CBD products are not checked by any authority!

There is therefore always the risk that the CBD products offered may be contaminated (contain toxins) or that the concentration indicated on the packaging does not correspond to reality.

Purity of CBD - what to consider!

The purity of CBD is an important issue.
The production of CBD products is not subject to any control!
Every seller and manufacturer advertise that their product is at least 99% pure.
But can such statements be believed?

Fact is: the purchase of pure, high-quality CBD oil is difficult!

The sale of CBD oil in pharmacies is prohibited in Germany, but not in Austria and Switzerland.
So, if you don't have a pharmacy as your first port of call for the purchase of high-quality, good and pure CBD oil, all you can do is shop online, or one or the other hemp shop.

But how can consumers be sure that they are also buying good quality?

A high price does not necessarily mean that the oil is clean and free of toxins. Also, the given % value does not really have to be correct!

On the CBD market there are now many black sheep!

Outside Europe, there are countries that have specialized in the cultivation of industrial hemp/utility hemp, in order to be able to cover the demand also in Europe.
But in these countries, there are no cultivation regulations.
Here, plants are often cultivated which already have a much higher basic value than is permitted in Germany, for example.

As mentioned before, in Germany only certified and approved farmers are allowed to grow certain varieties of useful hemp.
This lays a small foundation of safety for the consumer.

But one thing is certain: Using hemp from countries outside Europe poses a lot of health risks. It is absolutely undetectable how the hemp "grows up".
Are fertilizers, pesticides, herbicides used?
They represent the greatest danger.
Because a CBD contaminated with toxins is extremely dangerous to health!

As Germany is very strict with laws please – wherever – you are, be careful with buying CBD products!

How can a buyer of CBD products be sure to buy a good, pure product?

There are manufacturers/producers who document the origin and production of CBD products very precisely (HempWorx, Hemptouch and Cibidol keep very precise documentation).
The only advice to the consumer/buyer can be: allow enough time for the research and compare different suppliers exactly!
Providers who don't offer any documentation certainly have something to

hide!

The clearer and more detailed the production documentation is, if the origin of the processed hemp is not concealed, the safer it is to purchase a good and pure product.

Pure, good CBD products will have their price, but that should be worth your own health and safety!

There are also really black sheep whose products contain a much lower value or no CBD at all!

An example from the USA:

"The US Food and Drug Administration (FDA) conducted a comprehensive review of the various offers on the market in both 2015 and 2016.

It turned out that many suppliers made false claims regarding the concentration of the CBD in their oils.

Especially the faulty documentation between CBD and CBDA was decisive here.

While the effect of CBD has been very well researched, CBDA appears to be much less potent in its efficacy.

An agent that specifies a purity content of 5 % but is composed of 3.8 % CBD and 1.2 % CBDA cannot have the same effect as an oil with 5 % CBD."

7 WHICH CBD PRODUCTS ARE AVAILABLE FOR SALE?

In recent years, more and more CBD products have also come onto the market.

Here is a first overview:
- CBD Lip Care
- CBD Oils
- CBD Pastes
- CBD Teas
- CBD E-Liquids
- CBD Creams (for Psoriasis)
- CBD Creams (for eczema)
- CBD Creams (for acne)
- CBD Drops & melatonin (better sleep)
- CBD Capsules
- CBD Oil for Cats & Dogs
- CBD feeding supplement for cats & dogs
- …

8 CBD OIL CONCENTRATIONS AND RIGHT DOSAGE

CBD oil concentrations

If you read up on CBD oils online, you will quickly notice that they are available in different concentrations.

The most common concentrations are 2 %, 5 % and 10 %.
The higher the concentration, the more expensive the product.

The best way to "touch" CBD is to start with a low concentration.
If the low potent CBD oils have no or hardly any effect, the next step is to increase to the 5 % variant.
There can be no clear guideline, as every body reacts differently to CBD.

However, the higher the CBD concentration, the greater the effect.

There are manufacturers who offer CBD oil in the range up to 20%.
CBD pastes are available with 30 %, 40 % and 50 %.

How to use CBD and how to find the right dosage?
CBD is safe as a natural plant remedy.
Important: it must not contain any toxins!

Finding the right daily dose requires help and guidance, as there are some important factors in determining the right dose:
> Health condition/problem
> Intensity of the problem

- ➤ Personal metabolism
- ➤ Personal body chemistry
- ➤ What is the respective reaction to CBD?
- ➤ Cannabis Sensitivity
- ➤ Body weight
- ➤ Medications that are taken

It is best to start with a low dosage, which is then gradually increased as needed.
This enables the body to adapt gradually.

<u>Micro Dose</u>
The micro dose is often used for stress, sleep disorders, mood disorders, headaches, PTSD, nausea and metabolic disorders.

0.5 - 20 mg CBD/dose/day

Here the 5 % CBD oil is recommended.
1 drop is a quantity of about 1.6 mg CBD (always a little depending on the pipette used).
In this case, the revenue would be as follows:
3 drops 3x/day = approx. 15 mg

Standard Dose
The standard dose can be used for inflammation, pain, Lyme disease, autoimmune diseases, depression, anxiety, multiple sclerosis, fibromyalgia, autism, IBS, arthritis and to support weight loss.

10 mg - 100 mg CBD/dose/day

For the standard dose 15 % or 20 % CBD oil is suitable.
Depending on the pipette size, a tropical contains about 5 mg (15 %) or about 6.5 mg (20 %) CBD.

Recommended dosage:
CBD Oil 15 % = 3 drops 3x/day = approx. 45 mg CBD
CBD oil 20 % = 3 drops 3x/day = approx. 60 mg CBD
 = 6 drops 3x/day = approximately 120 mg CBD

Therapeutic Dose
In the therapeutic field one speaks of a high dose.
This is at a daily dose of 50 mg - 800 mg CBD/day.

Such a dose can only have a supporting effect in the area of the following clinical pictures:
seizures, epilepsy, cancer, liver disease and other life-threatening conditions.

CBD pastes are suitable for such therapeutic dosages. They can carry a higher dosage of CBD:
30 % paste: 1 ml = 300 mg CBD
40 % paste: 1 ml = 400 mg CBD
50 % paste: 1 ml = 500 mg CBD

General Guidelines for dosage:
There is no one size for dosing CBD.
How high the dosage can or should be varies from person to person and depends on the factors already mentioned.
If you are not sure which dosage is the right one, it is advisable to ask a doctor or therapist.

"Less is more" is basically the motto of cannabis therapy.
If the desired result is not achieved with a high dose, it is advisable to reduce the dose.
This is the easiest way to find out the personal best dose.
The results should also be monitored with the dose found in this way.
It may be necessary to increase the dose slightly after a certain period of time.

Please be patient, finding the right dose is essential but it may take a little while!

Important: if you are already taking certain medications, you must pay attention to possible side effects and/or interactions!

Taking CBD
CBD is best placed under the tongue.
You stand in front of the mirror.
This allows you to check that the drop is placed correctly.
Raise the tongue and use the pipette to drop the selected number of CBD drops centrally under the tongue into the palate.
Close your mouth - but don't swallow the CBD oil yet.
Within approx. 1 -2 minutes the oil is absorbed by the body (absorbed through the oral mucosa).
After that you swallow the rest
This is the fastest way to get the CBD into the bloodstream.

If you don't like the taste of CBD oil in your mouth, you can swallow it directly.
With this type of absorption (via the gastric mucosa), however, it takes longer until it reaches the brain via the blood.

The bottle should be well shaken before use, so that the active substances bind again well with the oil.

For better shelf life, CBD oil should be stored in a cool, dark place.
Nothing stands in the way of storage in the refrigerator.
The CBD oil should be at room temperature when ingested.

If a CBD paste is used, it is supplied with an applicator.
This allows the paste to be optimally placed under the tongue.

Tip:
Meanwhile different manufacturers offer the CBD oil also with taste (e.g. peppermint).

Please: if you are unsure seek the help of a professional!

Dosage mentioned here is the result of research !

Every person and every body is different and may react different.

The author is not responsible for incorrect individual intake.
The values given here are only a first guideline!

9 CBD THERAPY FOR SOME DISEASES

As already mentioned, there are some clinical pictures in which CBD has long been used as a therapeutic aid.

This has been the case in the USA for several years now, and more detailed information is already available.

These, however, come purely from users themselves or from the experience reports of accompanying therapists (doctors, naturopaths, alternative practitioners, homeopaths, ...).

CBD for migraine

Although people have been trying for many years to find the causes of migraines, they have still not been able to find them.

This circumstance makes a treatment of migraine patients also very difficult. It is suspected that genes play a role in migraine, as migraine occurs quite frequently within families.

It is also suspected that this is a so-called neurotransmitter disorder in the brain, usually in connection with reduced blood circulation.

Migraine is a pulsating headache that usually occurs only on one side of the head.

The migraine pain almost always increases with walking, head bending and movement.

The pain intensity is highest around the eye.

Migraine attacks last between 4 and 72 hours and are accompanied by nausea, vomiting and sensitivity to light.

Many sufferers report perception problems such as dizziness and visual problems before migraine breaks out (= aura).

All this has a lasting effect on the daily life and quality of life of migraine patients.

As an unaffected person, one is not aware that there are many different types of migraine.

Migraine also occurs in various forms:

➢ **auraless**
   this is the most common form.
   It occurs as a headache attack, with moderate to severe pain that increases with movement and lasts up to 72 hours.

➢ **with aura**
   about 30 % of all migraine patients report neurological symptoms before the migraine "hits" them
   o   malaise
   o   language difficulties
   o   fake
   o   visual disturbances such as flickering, seeing jagged lines, flashes of light
   o   skin sensation

After 30 - 60 minutes these complaints disappear again. The cause is suspected to be reduced blood circulation in the brain.

These aura symptoms can also be mistaken for the symptoms of an Imminent stroke.
But: In a migraine, the aura begins insidiously and then increases in intensity.
A stroke usually comes suddenly and without warning.
In case of doubt, a CT or MRT can determine exactly whether it is a migraine or a stroke.

➢ **Migraine myocardial infarction**
   If the aura symptoms persist for longer than 60 minutes, there may be a pronounced reduced blood circulation in individual areas of the brain. Such a lack of blood circulation is not harmless, as it can lead to permanent damage.
   Here, too, a CT or MRT can provide precise information.

➢ **Migralepsy**
   Migralepsy is also a consequence of a migraine attack with aura and is an epileptic seizure.
   It occurs during or within one hour after the migraine attack.

➢ ***Aura without headache***
It may happen that an aura occurs without the following headache.
This condition is colloquially referred to as eye migraine or migraine without headache.
This condition occurs in about 10% of classic migraine patients.
<u>Attention:</u> Here a thorough clarification is advisable, since such symptoms can rank among the first signs of a stroke!

➢ ***Vestibular Migraine***
The balance system is particularly affected here (dizziness and balance disorders).
The attack-like disturbance of the balance is in the foreground, a headache is also noticeable.
The symptoms are similar to those of Meunière's disease.

➢ ***Hemiplegic migraine = complicated migraine***
It is rather rare but occurs more frequently in the family.
In addition to the other known migraine symptoms, there is the limitation of movement.
It is extremely difficult for patients to move certain limbs in a targeted manner.
Sometimes a movement is not possible at all.
After approx. 1 hour these symptoms usually disappear again.
This is suspected of a genetic defect on the 1st, 2nd and 19th chromosomes.

➢ ***Basilar migraine***
This is also a subtype of migraine with aura.
Mostly young adults are affected, and the headache is increasingly in the back of the head.
It is assumed that the arteria basilaris (supplies the cerebellum and the brain stem with blood) temporarily cramps.
This leads to a temporary undersupply of these areas and manifests itself with various symptoms:
- o motor coordination disorder
- o speech disorder
- o dizziness, tinnitus, hearing loss
- o Visual disturbances (double vision, visual field deficits, ...)
- o disturbance of consciousness
- o sensitive sensations (on both sides)

➢ *LiS (Locked in Syndrome)*
Very rarely, LiS occurs as a result of basilar migraine.
The affected person is fully conscious but can no longer communicate or move.
This condition can last between 2 and 30 minutes.

➢ *Migraine of the eyes (retinal or opthalmoplegic migraine)*
Retinal: very rare special form in children and adolescents.
About 1 hour before the onset of headache, visual field deficits, visual disturbances (flickering in front of the eyes) and temporary blindness occur.
They disappear as soon as the headache sets in
Opthalmoplegic: Extremely rare!
It affects both eyes at the same time and manifests itself as a visual disturbance.
Due to their rarity, physicians are not sure whether this condition can be classified as migraine or as another disease!

➢ *Menstrual migraine*
It occurs exclusively with menstruation, approximately 2 days before and up to 2 days after menstruation.
The symptoms are those of a "normal" migraine, but more intense and prolonged.
About 7% of all women suffer from it. The cause is assumed to be a sharp drop in oestrogen levels.

➢ *Hormonally Conditioned Migraine*
Here migraine attacks occur not only in connection with menstruation, but also during the cycle.

➢ *Chronic migraine*
If a patient has migraine attacks on more than 15 days/month and for more than 3 months, it is called chronic migraine.
Even the time between attacks is not free of complaints.

➢ *Abdominal migraine*
This is a special form and mostly affects children.
The pain focuses on the area around the navel and can occur along with nausea and vomiting, loss of appetite and pallor. An accompanying headache is rare. An attack can last from 1 hour to several days.
The causes are still in the dark.
Affected children must be able to rest and relax!

Children suffering from abdominal migraine very often get a classic migraine as adults.

> ### ➢ *Migraine in childhood*
> If migraine already occurs in childhood, headache is usually bilateral in the forehead and temples.
> As pure headache is often absent in children, migraine is not recognised here.
> Accompanying symptoms: balance disorders, dizziness and sensitivity to odours.
> A child can often not describe the symptoms correctly.
> Persistent or more frequently acute symptoms such as fatigue, apathy, paleness, dizziness, nausea and vomiting, but abdominal pains are often signs.
> Psychological (school, conflicts, quarrels) and/or physical (exhaustion, fatigue, drinking too little or eating too little) stress is often the main cause of migraine in children.
> <u>Difficulty</u>: With children, drug therapy often does not work very well.
> This is why we focus on non-drug therapy: regular daily routine, biofeedback, learning relaxation methods, ...

Once you have received all this migraine information, you ask yourself:
If regular medication can't help migraine patients enough, how can CBD help?
Due to the lack of scientific knowledge - once again - you can only orient yourself on the experiences of therapists or on the experience reports of those affected themselves.

Migraine patients are often desperate when drug therapy cannot help.
Because migraine means a very great reduction in the quality of life.
For this reason alone, migraine patients have always been on the lookout for alternative ways to better tolerate the migraine phase.
It is often read that CBD is a miracle cure for migraine.
Whether this is really the case can be answered badly.
It is a fact, however, that a large number of migraine patients who have been taking CBD oil for many years have found a remedy that makes migraines more bearable.

One patient reports that she has been carrying 5% CBD oil in her handbag for some time now.
As she is often exposed to stress situations at work and these often trigger a

migraine, she has already tried to drip 1 - 2 CBD drops into her mouth at the onset of stress.

She could quickly notice a calming of her nerves and relax.

Encouraged by this, she then applied a few drops of CBD oil to her tongue at the first signs of migraine and allowed it to act through the oral mucosa.

The pain disappeared a short time later and the migraine did not break out!

For the first time in a 15-year history of suffering, this woman has been able to prevent a massive migraine outbreak with CBD.

In addition, the despair and stress ("now I have this stupid migraine again") is not at all pronounced and the general condition is much calmer and more relaxed.

A pharmacist who himself offers CBD products in his pharmacy has described the possible effect on his migraine patients:

- ➢ CBD relieves pain
- ➢ The cannabidiol is believed to block pain receptors in the brain. This prevents the transmission of pain.
- ➢ As a result, the sensitivity to pain decreases
- ➢ CBD has an anti-inflammatory effect and protects the nerves.
- ➢ By the additional intake of CBD with migraine, conventional painkillers can be reduced
- ➢ It does not lead to any dependency
- ➢ CBD also regulates the serotonin level (serotonin = happiness hormone, regulates mood and emotion)
- ➢ Serotonin also plays a central role in the sensation of pain (it controls nausea and vomiting).
- ➢ It has been proven that the serotonin level in migraine is subject to very large fluctuations:
    - o before the seizure it rises sharply
    - o after the seizure, the value is extremely low

  The blood vessels dilate when not enough serotonin is available and the inflammatory and pain inducing substances enter the brain much more easily.
- ➢ CBD regulates the release of serotonin, keeps it relatively stable (so the values remain in balance)

Through CBD, a large number of migraine patients receive a better quality of life again!

Cannabis in Pain Therapy

As already mentioned, there are some clinical pictures in which CBD has long been used as a therapeutic aid.

This has been the case in the USA for several years now, and more detailed information is already available.

These, however, come purely from users themselves or from the experience reports of accompanying therapists (doctors, naturopaths, alternative practitioners, homeopaths, ...).

CBD and Autism

Parents of autistic children and autistic adults still have a hard time in our society.

Hardly anyone knows that there are different forms of autism.

3 forms of autism:
> Early childhood autism
> Atypical autism
> Asperger's syndrome
>

In all 3 autism forms almost the same disturbances occur
> disruption of communication (verbal and non-verbal)
> conspicuous behaviour patterns such as constraints (repeatedly counting objects, ...)
> considerable difficulties in social interaction

Autism cannot be cured at the present time because the causes of this congenital disease have not yet been clarified.

For this reason, there are also no drugs that promise help.

Parents of autistic children try everything to make their children's lifes as good as possible and are always looking for alternative methods to help their children.

The use of CBD in autism is smiled at by orthodox medicine.

Not so from concerned parents.

They are very open to CBD, especially because the experience reports are very positive.

Irrespective of gender and age, autistic people are much more open and emotionally alert when treated with CBD.

As a result, the willingness to approach people - to act with them and to perceive their social environment better - increases.

It may not be much at first glance, but for the parents and families of autistic people and also for the autistic people themselves, it means a lot.

What do affected people or parents say about the use of CBD?

"I am also an Asperger autist and I have found that under the influence of cannabis I have much higher social skills, can have conversations and understand fellow human beings."

"Of course, healing is probably not possible.
However, the symptoms can be significantly alleviated.
One theory for the development of autism is a disturbance in the body's own ECS (endocannabinoid system).
Therefore, it is understandable that added cannabinoids start exactly where the problem originally arose."

<u>CBD for Multiple Sclerosis</u>

Multiple sclerosis falls into the group of neurological autoimmune diseases and affects the central nervous system (CNS).
Young adults and middle-aged people are the most frequently affected.
It is very different for each patient.
What this disease always brings with it, however, is a gradual weakening of the body.
Incapacity to work often occurs very quickly. Also, multiple sclerosis patients are often very quickly dependent on care and help.
There are slow, creeping courses of disease, but also those where so-called relapses occur (sudden severe deterioration of the state of health).

Symptoms like
> paralyzing muscle cramps
> palsies
> less and less mobility due to stiff limbs
> aches
> blisters functional disorders
> seeing, hearing, tasting, smelling and sense of balance are increasingly disturbed.
> Spasticity (= excessive tension of the skeletal muscles (cause: damage to the spinal cord and/or brain))

increasingly affect the quality of life of MS patients.

Multiple sclerosis is also still one of the diseases that cannot be cured!
From a medical therapeutic point of view, medication has so far only been able to slow down the course of the disease.
The earlier MS is diagnosed, the better the chances of success.

How can CBD now be used in MS therapy?
Due to the properties of CBD, pain tolerance can be improved in the area of

multiple sclerosis-related pain.
Less pain in the limbs means better mobility.
CBD also has an anti-inflammatory effect.
Since many multiple sclerosis patients often become depressed as a result of all their symptoms and the fact that MS is incurable, CBD can also help here. Experiences of MS patients who have been using CBD regularly for some time have all reported a noticeable reduction in spasms (due to the antispasmodic properties of CBD).

Dosage for supportive treatment of Multiple Sclerosis:
Well, this question cannot simply be answered with a CBD product and a daily dose.
As mentioned earlier, every patient is different.
The course of MS is different and of course every human body is different.
What the findings in CBD therapy of MS patients in recent years have shown, however, is that an effect starts at a daily dose of approximately 25 mg CBD. If a patient suffers from very severe symptoms, such a dosage can be carefully increased within a week.
In this area, however, it is always advisable to seek the advice of an experienced therapist in this area and also to agree to monitoring the dosage in your own interest.

It can be administered with CBD oil, paste or by inhalation (e-cigarette).

If you are an MS patient and would like to learn more about MS and CBD, I recommend the book by Elizabeth Limbach.
Having contracted MS over 20 years ago, she discovered CBD in search of help and relief and summarized all her experiences in the book "Cannabis Saved-My-Life".

CBD and Cancer
For many people, the diagnosis of cancer is still one of the most frightening. Although there are some types of cancer that are well treatable and curable, there are also those that are still a death sentence.
But not only the disease itself, but also the often highly invasive forms of treatment (radiation, chemotherapy, etc.) demand a lot from the already very weakened bodies of cancer patients.
In recent years, more and more cancer patients have placed their trust in CBD as a complementary treatment.
Unfortunately, there are only animal studies in this area so far, but these are promising:
Animal studies have shown that CBD can inhibit the growth of some cancer

cells (leukemia, cervical and prostate cancer, breast cancer).
The effect of CBD on cancer cells of the nervous system (neuroblastoma) has also been investigated and there are positive approaches.
Neuroblastoma is the most common cause of childhood malignant cancer.

A study in cancer patients (brain tumor and breast cancer) came to the conclusion that already at a dose of 20 mg synthetic cannabidiol (drug!) an effect sets in.
The conclusion of the authors of this study is as follows:

"Cannabidiol is a potential candidate for the therapy especially of patients with breast cancer or glioblastoma. Especially when conventional therapy has been unsuccessful. Important: CBD is not an alternative to conventional cancer therapy for breast cancer and glioblastomas and all other forms of cancer. Further studies investigating the effect of CBD on cancer patients are desirable to better evaluate the effect of CBD as a potential cancer drug. "

As already mentioned, health insurance companies often cover the costs of cannabinoids (drugs) for tumor pain and nausea as a result of radiation and chemotherapy.
However, it is also worth making an application to cover the costs of cannabidiols (CBD). There is a good chance that the costs will be covered, especially in the case of severe disease progressions, although neither CBD nor THC are recognized as cancer drugs.
It is best to discuss the dosage and the appropriate CBD preparation with a doctor, who must also prescribe it so that the application can be approved by the health insurance company.

CBD and Diabetes

Diabetes is a widespread disease today.
At least one in five Germans is already suffering from diabetes.
Approximately 90% suffer from type 2 diabetes.
Children and adolescents are also increasingly affected.
In the USA, the number of diabetes patients is even higher. (2015: 22,4 million diagnosed diabetes patients and around 7,2 million still undiagnosed!)
This is also the reason why researchers and doctors in the USA are very active in research.
Cannabidiol-containing products and CBD oil are now regarded as a possible solution.
In summary, 5 important findings are reported:
    1) For several years, a group of people at risk for type 2 diabetes who had not yet developed diabetes was examined, treated and

accompanied.
In this "preliminary stage" the "patients" already very often have an insulin resistance and a far elevated fasting insulin level, as well as a remarkably low cholesterol (lipoprotein) content.
Results of the 5-year study:
- o with regular use of cannabis/hemp =
- o 16% lower insulin levels with regular use of cannabis/hemp
- o 17 % lower insulin resistance
- o higher content of lipoprotein cholesterol

2) Insulin resistance is an important criterion in both type 2 and prediabetes.
It is like a cycle: body cells reject insulin, but they can no longer absorb the glucose they need for their energy.
Glucose decomposes directly in the bloodstream = high blood sugar levels.
How exactly CBD helps here is still a little unclear, but:
- o CBD has a very strong anti-inflammatory effect.
- o here a connection is seen (chronic inflammations with insulin resistance)
- o fewer inflammations improve the immune system in general, but also cell growth and sugar metabolism in particular

3) Overweight as a risk factor
It has been proven by research that CBD affects body functions, which in turn plays a role in weight control.
- o it acts as an appetite suppressant (overeating, weight gain)
- o it reduces weight by combating inflammation
- o it helps the body to use/burn calories more effectively

4) Nerve damage in hands and feet is often the result of diabetes. These are accompanied by pain, tingling and numbness. This area is still being researched, but it is believed that CBD
- o helps to relieve pain
- o prevents new nerve damage
- o can increase nerve growth
- o protects the liver from oxidative stress

5) Another consequence of diabetes is skin damage, open wounds that are difficult to heal, ... Cannabis oil (also in ointments!) helps with
- o itching
- o other skin irritations
- o burning
- o ...

The irritated and affected skin areas usually react very quickly to the anti-inflammatory and moisturising properties of CBD oil.

CBD for Weight Loss

Since just the weight loss with CBD support was addressed, we give you some additional information.

Obesity - Obesity is still on the rise in our industrialized countries.

Since overweight is also associated with diseases such as high blood pressure, diabetes, sleep apnea, breathing difficulties, movement restrictions, ..., overweight means less quality of life.

However, losing the weight that has been gained is a challenge.

"What I've eaten little by little can't go away overnight!"

Sufficient exercise and a healthy, clean diet are the basis for healthy weight loss.

Diets and pills (often with many side effects) that promise miracles are expensive and don`t bring miracles!

CBD is not a miracle cure for weight loss either, but it can support you very well:

> CBD suppresses ravenous appetite
> CBD curbs appetite
> CBD has a very positive influence on fat burning and metabolism.
> CBD increases the number of mitochondria (important for fat reduction)
> CBD "blocks" proteins produced by fat cells (less new fat is added)

A CBD oil with 5 % or 10 % is recommended to support weight loss. A general dosage instruction cannot be given here either.

However, the start is often recommended:

- 5 drops 5 % CBD oil per day
- Body observation
- possibly adjust the dose a little more

make sure to pay attention to the quality of the CBD oil!

CBD and Crohn's disease

Crohn's disease is an inflammatory bowel disease that causes inflammation throughout the digestive tract.

This leads to severe abdominal pain and diarrhea.

For the patients, the disease is very tiring and also very painful.

The result is rapid weight loss and even malnutrition.

Even this disease is not curable until today!

Within orthodox medicine remains only the pain therapy, in order to make the life of the patients a little more pleasant.

CBD is usually used as a supplement.

On the one hand to alleviate the inflammations and on the other hand to support the pain relief.

In contrast to the strong painkillers used in pharmaceutical medicine, CBD is almost free of side effects (see CBD and its side effects).

Children and elderly people suffering from Crohn's disease can also be treated with CBD. In addition to CBD oil, CBD capsules or chewable tablets are particularly suitable.

With regard to a given dosage recommendation, the same applies as always to CBD:

- each body reacts differently
- 25 mg CBD/day is effective in most people
- only increase the dosage slowly if the symptoms are severe
- observe well
- in case of doubt ask a doctor or therapist for advice

Experiences of patients suffering from Crohn's disease:

"...has been diagnosed with Crohn's disease and has confirmed that CBD has done much to alleviate nausea and pain. When he was diagnosed with the disease, the medication prescribed by the doctor was a little helpful, only that he felt sick and depressed after taking it. The CBD oil, however, has already achieved good results after only a few weeks "

"... is another patient who has been taking CBD oil for Crohn's disease for three weeks and says that the symptoms no longer occur. He takes the drops once a day and the results are amazing. He is even able to eat regularly without vomiting. "

CBD application in children

As promising as the experiences and reports on the application of CBD are in many areas, the question arises for parents of sick children, for example: Can I help my child with CBD?

CBD for children is legal to buy.

But here, too, the note applies: the effect of CBD on children has NOT been scientifically proven.

Cannabidiole ingredients that are important and good for children:

- ➤ the oil is rich in vitamins B1, B2, E
- ➤ It has a high content of minerals such as calcium, potassium, magnesium, iron, copper, sodium, zinc, phosphorus.
- ➤ also valuable proteins are contained
- ➤ it is characterised by a high proportion of essential fatty acids (omega 3 and omega 6)

> gamma linolenic acid is also included

CBD oil can help with a variety of different conditions in children, but as already mentioned it is not a miracle cure.

It can be taken pure and undiluted.

Since the taste of the CBD does not necessarily appeal to every child, it is also possible to add the CBD drops to fatty foods. This makes it easier for the children to digest.

In a nutshell:

> CBD is applicable to children
> studies and field reports confirm good results in the treatment of epilepsy in children
> CBD helps children suffering from sleep disorders, anxiety and general restlessness.
> it relaxes
> with ADHD it can easily be integrated into the everyday life of the children with the aim to reduce or completely avoid treatment with Ritalin
> it makes sense to discuss the use of CBD with your pediatrician and to seek advice on the correct dosage.
> ss the parents of a child diagnosed with ADHD, you can also talk to your doctor about CBD without hesitation, especially if you are looking for an alternative to Ritalin, which is controversial because of its many and often strong side effects.

The results associated with long-term CBD use are also quite astonishing for many other diseases.

In this area it would be desirable if CBD were also taken more seriously by science and orthodox medicine and if concrete results from corresponding studies could be consulted in the coming years. Such results would certainly be helpful, especially in the area of minimum and maximum dosages. But it would also increase the general acceptance of CBD.

10 SIDE EFFECT AND SOME ADDITIONAL INFORMATION ABOUT CBD

SIDE EFFECTS OF CBD

In general, it can be said that CBD has very few side effects.

From the little what is known:

<u>Short-term side effect:</u>
lightheadedness
dry mouth
fatigue
diarrhoea
decrease/increase of appetite

<u>Long-term side effects:</u>
none known yet

It is not recommended to take CBD during pregnancy.
So far, it is only known that CBD affects some proteins that also play an important role in placental function.
Since it is suspected that the placenta may not function properly as a result and problems may arise during pregnancy, it is better to avoid CBD during pregnancy.

SOME ADDITIONAL INFORMATION ABOUT CBD

CBD E-Liquid
As mentioned earlier, CBD enters the bloodstream and the brain very quickly via the lungs.
When inhaling CBD oil, it is difficult to dose correctly.
In recent years, e-cigarettes have established themselves on the market and even CBD producers have recognized the chance of a market share.

CBD oils that are suitable for oral consumption cannot be used in e-cigarettes!

The CBD E-Liquids are accordingly manufactured without oil (oil must not be inhaled!).

By using an e-cigarette, the liquids are only vaporized by heating for a long time. There are no harmful substances as they are produced during combustion (cigarette).
CBD e-liquids should always be transparent.
There should also be a homogeneous liquid in the vial (no substances should settle from each other).
Meanwhile, various manufacturers offer CBD liquids with different flavors (peppermint, strawberry, mango, blueberry, ...).
The CBD % share in the e-liquids also varies.

IMPORTANT: When purchasing, make sure that the THC content in the CBD E-Liquid does not exceed 0.2 %!

<u>Advantages and disadvantages of CBD E-Liquids:</u>
Advantages
positive effect on the immune system
helpful in: mental and physical ailments
Taste can be varied
Calming in stressful situations

Drawback
Not usable without e-cigarette

When buying e-liquids, it is worth doing a little research and comparing.
Important:
Ingredients (E 1520, E 422, distilled water, natural flavours)
Dosage (50 mg - 1000 mg)
Quantity (sales size is usually 10ml)
Taste (other flavourings)
Effect (faster effect than oils and tablets; possible seconds after inhalation)
As far as dosage is concerned, you should know: the higher the dosage, the better the positive effect on body and mind!

Travelling with CBD products

<u>CBD E-Liquids</u>
Basically, travelling with CBD E-Liquids is not a problem.
Within Europe, care should be taken that the maximum THC value is not higher than 0.0199 %.
The situation is different for trips to the USA.
E-cigarettes are allowed in hand luggage and also filled with a CBD E-Liquid.
Now the big BUT:
The CBD E-Liquid should always contain 0 % THC.
The reason for this is first of all the strict control at the entry, on the other hand also the very different regulation in the individual federal states of the USA.
If you travel with a 0% CBD E-Liquid, you can travel to any state in the USA without thinking about it.

Tip:
Carry the manufacturer's certificate of composition and THC content (trustworthy manufacturers can always be found on the website).
If not, request this from the manufacturers).

In general, it can be said that travelling with CBD products within the Schengen countries should be possible without hesitation if you stick to the 0.2% border.
If you travel outside the Schengen area, the country-specific CBD limits must be observed.
In case of doubt, always carry written product information (in local language or English) with you.

If you travel to a country where the cultivation, consumption and sale of cannabis products with a THC content are prohibited, you should NOT carry your CBD products with you!

<u>Here are some current country information:</u>
USA
CBD oils are legalized in many states, but the regulations regarding ingredients and permitted quantities vary from state to state and must be observed.
Active substance limits are to be observed in:
Alabama, Georgia, Indiana, Iowa, Kentucky, Louisiana, Mississippi, Missouri, North Carolina, Oklahoma, South Carolina, Tennessee, Texas, Utah, Virginia, Wisconsin, Wyoming, Florida and Idaho.
New York and California have further legalizations of THC
Canada
In Canada, CBD products with a THC content of up to 0.3% may be sold and consumed without medical prescription.

If reliable and up-to-date information on the legality of CBD products and maximum limits is needed, this can be obtained promptly (often at short notice) from the embassies or consulates of the respective countries.

In addition to the ingredients and % values, the import quantity is also important to consider.
As a rule of thumb, however, this is the case in most countries: Cosmetics and medication for the duration of the stay/journey may be carried.
Please think of the 100 ml limit in your hand luggage.

CBD COMPACT

CBD is not a miracle cure!

But: it can be used in many areas of health and thus at least bring relief and improvement to people with health problems.

The consumer is also responsible for taking CBD:

It is your duty to inform yourself about the composition of the CBD product, its origin and the ingredients.

This is necessary because the manufacture and trade of CBD products in Germany is not subject to any controls.

CBD is not a medical product and the purchase takes place almost exclusively via the Internet or hemp shops.

In Germany CBD cannot be bought in pharmacies.

In Austria and Switzerland there are now pharmacies which offer CBD and other hemp products (here the legal situation is different from in Germany). Every country handles this very different.

In the USA every state has its own laws.

Due to the fact that the majority of the market is on the Internet, there are unfortunately more and more "black sheep".

But once you have played it safe, clarified all relevant points and found a CBD product you can trust, you will soon discover that CBD can have a positive effect on many diseases.

Migraine patients who have been struggling with these uncontrollable headaches for many years or even their whole lives, for whom normal painkillers do not help well or not at all, should try using CBD oil in addition. The experience reports of those affected give great hope that the migraine will at least become more bearable, or that it will not break out in the first place.

This fact alone means an important improvement in the quality of life for migraine patients.

But in addition to the treatment of migraine, there are a large number of other conditions where CBD brings relief:

- ➢ Autism
- ➢ Alzheimer/Dementia
- ➢ Arthrosis
- ➢ Arthritis
- ➢ Overload/sStress
- ➢ Insomnia
- ➢ Acne

- ➢ Diabetes
- ➢ Asthma and Allergies
- ➢ Cancer
- ➢ Epilepsy
- ➢ Multiple Sclerosis
- ➢ Crohn's Disease
- ➢ Fibromyalgie
- ➢ Smoking Cessation
- ➢ Addiction Disorders
- ➢ Rheumatism
- ➢ Sepsis
- ➢ Hepatitis
- ➢ Nausea
- ➢ Overweight/Obesity
- ➢ …

For some of these clinical pictures it is absolutely advisable to arrange an additional treatment with CBD with the treating physician.
On the one hand to rule out interactions with already prescribed medications, but also to find the right dosage for each individual case.

CBD products are now also offered in forms other than just CBD oil.
This has also broadened the range of possible applications.
CBD oil is available in various grades up to a concentration of 20 %.
If a higher dosage is required, CBD pastes are recommended.
CBD pastes can be concentrated up to 50 % CBD.
If you don't like the taste of CBD in drop form very much, you can now also use CBD capsules or CBD chewable tablets.
Some manufacturers now also offer CBD oil with flavors (peppermint, fruit flavors, ...).

The best way to deliver CBD to the body is orally. Put the required number of drops in the middle of the tongue and let them work for 1 to 2 minutes through the mucous membrane of the mouth until you swallow them. In this way, the ingredients reach the blood relatively quickly.

CBD has no serious side effects (only known as interaction with drugs).
Even an overdose has not yet really occurred.
In the therapeutic field, doses of up to 800 mg CBD/day can be used without any problems.

However, "less is often more" is a good guideline for taking CBD.
When you start taking CBD, it is wise to start with a low dosage first.

If the desired effect does not occur, the dosage can be gradually increased until relief occurs.

If, for example, you take a relatively high dose in the case of migraine and do not notice any change, it is advisable to gradually reduce the dosage. In this way, the optimum dosage can be found quickly.

Why is there no dosage information for CBD?

The correct dosage of CBD varies from person to person and depends on:
- Health condition or problem
- Intensity of the problem
- Personal metabolism
- personal body chemistry
- What is the reaction to CBD?
- Cannabis Sensitivity
- body weight
- Medications that are taken

High quality CBD products are not cheap.

In Germany, the cultivation of useful hemp plants is regulated by law and only authorized farmers may plant certain varieties under specified conditions.

This gives a certain security for CBD products, which are produced from German hemp.

This is very important especially with regard to any harmful toxins that may be present.

Suspiciously cheap CBD products are often produced with hemp from non-European countries.

Here there are no regulations for the cultivation or use of pesticides, fertilizers, ...

CBD products made with such hemp may contain toxins or have a higher natural THC content.

If this is not properly and sufficiently "washed out" during production, such products may contain more THC and unwanted toxins than permitted.

Manufacturers who work with good hemp have nothing to hide and very often publish precise descriptions of their products (origin of the hemp, ingredients of the product, CBD content, ...).

If you travel outside Europe, e.g. USA, Canada, ... it always makes sense to carry a product certificate (preferably in English) with you.

Information about the legality of CBD in the respective holiday country can be obtained from the embassies and consulates of the holiday country.
The duty to inform lies here with the traveler!

Over the last few years, more and more CBD e-liquids have been coming onto the market.
If this is a high-quality, pure product, the inhalation of the vaporized (not burnt) CBD via the lungs is a way to quickly feel an effect.
The CBD passes through the lungs into the bloodstream and very quickly into the brain.
E-Liquids also have different concentrations and some manufacturers are now able to produce a completely THC-free CBD E-Liquid.
This can then be taken with you on journeys without any problems in your hand luggage.

To sum up:
CBD is not a miracle cure, although many sick people often use the term.
CBD can provide relief where conventional remedies and drugs do not work or do not work as well.
CBD products will never be a substitute for a prescribed drug, but the supportive effect in many areas can be demonstrated by many testimonials.
For the future, it is certainly desirable that there should be more scientific studies dealing with the respective modes of action of CBD.

As a complementary treatment to most clinical pictures, the costs of CBD therapy are not paid for by health insurance companies.
This can mean a high financial burden for the chronically ill.
However, cancer patients have a chance to receive financial support from health insurance companies.
Any chronically ill person who can be helped with CBD under medical supervision should, with the assistance of their doctor, try to apply to their health insurance company for reimbursement.

Conclusion: You should give CBD a chance and try it out.
Perhaps it will bring exactly the relief/improvement that you have been looking for for so long.
Then CBD will be your personal miracle cure.

ABOUT THE AUTHOR

FlyGirl is a passionate rider, loves to spend time with her friends in Texas every year.
After raising 3 kids on her own and often just working different jobs to pay the bills and to survive, she decided in 2019 to start writing again, because writing is her passion and she just loves it.

When she talks about her kids she has a smile on her face because she is proud that her "clan" is growing with a first daughter in law and a 1 year young granddaughter and another grandchild on the way, and more growth to come in the future.

There will be more from her in the future. Some books like her first Wind Therapy, a book about female riders worldwide, others like this one about CBD or Intermittent Fastening, ….
All her books can be found on Amazon.

THANK YOU

To Jenn Kulick.

She is my riding sister from Bandera/Texas and she is responsible for my cover designs.
But she is also an amazing photographer and much more.
Check out her portfolio
https://wildcreekink.co/

DISCLAIMER

The implementation of all information, instructions and strategies contained in this book is at your own risk. The author cannot assume any liability for any damages of any kind for any legal reason. Liability claims regarding damage caused by the use of any information provided, including any kind of information which is incomplete or incorrect, will therefore be rejected. Any legal claims and claims for damages are therefore also excluded. This work has been written down with the greatest care to the best of our knowledge and belief. For the topicality, completeness and quality of the information the author takes over however no guarantee. Printing errors and false information can also not be completely excluded. No legal responsibility or liability in any form can be assumed for incorrect information provided by the author.

COPYRIGHT

Imprint:

© Flygirl

2020

1st edition

All rights reserved.

Reprinting, even in extracts, not permitted.

No part of this work may be reproduced or transmitted in any form or by any means, electronic, mechanical, photocopying, recording or otherwise without the written permission of the author.

be reproduced, duplicated or distributed in any form.

Contact: blue.fantasy.writing@gmail.com